Copyright © 2010 by Emn

Published by Emma O. Neg

All rights reserved. No part of this book may be reproduced in any form or by any electronic or mechanical means, including information storage or retrieval systems, without permission in writing by publisher. Scanning, uploading or electronic distribution of this book or the facilitation of such without the permission of the publisher is prohibited. Please purchase only authorized public editions and do not participate in or encourage electronic piracy of copyrighted materials. Your support of the author's rights is appreciated. Any member of educational institutions wishing to photocopy part or the entire book for classroom use, or anthology; should send inquiries to emmalita@hotmail.com.

Published and Printed in the United States of America

ISBN-13 978-1456304492

How I Do It

EMMA O. NEGRETE FITNESS HANDBOOK HOW I DO IT

How I Do It

Acknowledgement		5
Chapter One-	Identifying Any Health Factors	9
Chapter Two-	Mental Preparation for Making Fitness Your Lifestyle	14
Chapter Three-	Nutrition	17
Chapter Four-	Supplements	27
Chapter Five-	Stretching and Warming Up	31
Chapter Six-	Strength Training	35
Chapter Seven-	Cardiovascular Exercise	61
Chapter Eight-	Controlling Stress	66
Chapter Nine-	Overcoming an Injury	69
Chapter Ten-	Training for Endurance vs. Strength	74
Chapter Eleven-	Training Plateaus	79
Chapter Twelve-	Different Theories of Fat Storage	82
Chapter Thirteen-	Perimenopause Years - Keeping the Beauty & Sexy Alive	86
Chapter Fourteen-	Genetics - Fiber Type I or Type II	97
Chapter Fifteen-	Foods	100
Chapter Sixteen-	Handling Holiday Festivities	105
Glossary of Terms		108

How I Do It

ATTENTION: This book is informational only. The data and information contained herein are based upon information from personal experiences, various published as well as unpublished sources, merely represent training, health, and nutrition literature, and practice as summarized by the authors and editors. The publisher of this book makes no warranties, expressed or implied, regarding the currency, completeness or scientific accuracy of this information, nor does it warrant the fitness of the information for any particular purpose. The information is not intended for use in connection with the sale of any product. Any claims or presentations regarding any specific products are strictly the responsibility of the product owners and/or manufacturers. This summary of information is not intended to REPLACE THE ADVICE OR ATTENTION OF HEALTH CARE PROFESSIONALS. It is not meant to be a source of clinical advice in any sense of the word. It is not intended to direct behavior or replace independent professional judgment. If you have a problem with your health, or before you begin on any beauty, health, fitness, sport training or nutritional programs, seek the permission from a qualified health care professional.

How I Do It

ACKNOWLEDGEMENT

This book is written due to the vast inquiries on how I do it in order to continue my passion in fitness and age gracefully even through my initial years of perimenopause.

I have written this book for you all who have taken such interest in my fitness journey and have indicated that I have inspired you to be the best possible self. I began writing this book with the intention of sharing my mind, body and soul equilibrium and have found that I needed to dissect my writings into a few books in order to provide the best clarity in all the gifts that GOD has given me.

This book will tell you what and how I do it to stay in shape and feel good about my physical being on and through perimenopause. It will convey the variety of training I do, the supplements I take, what my nutrition planning is like; how I overcame my back injuries along with anti-aging products and rituals I do to live the way I am today. There are no intentions here to sell a product but rather to allow you the opportunity to explore what may seem to be best for you in your current stage in life.

In fact, I had started writing a fitness book a little over a decade when I was again inspired by fellow

How I Do It

friends and/or clients to put my knowledge in writing. However, due to time constraints, I was unable to continue those works.

Therefore, I am continuing my works and writing this book at the age of 47 years young and with as much compassion, warmth and love to you all.

Most importantly, I want you to enjoy this read and therefore I purposely have not congested it with definitions, photographs and/or charts. I want to convey as much information as possible without getting too scientific as that would, more than likely, be another book or books in themselves.

I pray that all who are reading this book will find it helpful, fulfilling and a joy to discover that life is about living the best possible self by taking control of YOU and your desires. May you put all your passions to use and allow your Higher Power to grant you more in the abundance of life.

I want to thank you, in advance, for purchasing this book on my fitness rituals and hope that you will find your love in fitness as I did over three decades ago.

Much Love Worldwide..Believe & Succeed!

E-

How I Do It

*Dedication to my Mother & Father,
Maria (Fita) & Gumercindo*

How I Do It

Be

Your

Best

Self

At

Any

Age

:o)!

How I Do It

Chapter One

IDENTIFYING ANY HEALTH FACTORS

Understanding the stages of your life is very important to achieving the best possible you. If you have an ailment and/or are being treated with medication, it is important to understand the side effects in order to properly supplement your nutrition plan along with performing the appropriate exercise. For example, if you suffer from stress/anxiety, it is important to get on the proper nutrition plan and/or possible medication in order to actually perform your activities of daily living (ADLs) that hopefully include an exercise program. In addition, you may also find that yoga itself may relieve stress and this suffices for you.

Whether it is your adolescent years or your adult years. Whether it is perimenopause or menopause. All these stages will affect your body in some way. You must understand what is causing your symptoms(cause & effect) that are occurring in your body in order to take the proper course of action. For instance, as I am in my perimenopausal years, I recognize that my diet will require more supplements (fish oil, B12, B6, fiber, calcium, vitamin C, vitamin D) in order to maintain the same stamina for performing my ADLs which include cardiovascular and weight-training activity. I

How I Do It

recognize that in order to not sabotage my workout plan and health, I must readjust my workout schedule when my stress levels are high.

Therefore, on months when my menstrual cycle is off and my body is under more unwanted stress, I break my workouts to cardiovascular and weight training separately. In fact, my weight training is with lower weights and higher repetition in order to reduce stress, which reduces cortisol levels; hence not contradicting or negating my workouts. High cortisol levels cause the body to retain more fat thus decreasing the muscle building process. This occurs because cortisol also reduces the utilization of amino acids for protein formation in muscle cells. A cortisol excess can lead to a progressive loss of protein, muscle weakness and atrophy, and loss of bone mass through increased calcium excretion and less calcium absorption. Excess cortisol can also adversely affect tendon health. Cortisol causes a redistribution of body fat to occur and therefore, the lower extremities lose fat and muscle while the midsection and face become fatter.

If possible, I also have added napping and/or resting during the day. During perimenopause, the body is going through major changes that require extra attention and care. In some cases, the severity of perimenopausal symptoms may require some form of medication in order to regain your quality of life.

How I Do It

Some women may opt for hormone therapy replacement. However, hormones are something I have not explored as of yet as I believe the body is in a natural state of influx between cycles and hormone levels will vary every month, hence; no real accuracy on how much of what hormone to take monthly. I may explore that avenue when I finally reach menopause and/or depending on my quality of life.

How I Do It

Notes

Believe

and

Succeed!

How I Do It

Chapter Two

MENTAL PREPARATION FOR MAKING FITNESS YOUR LIFESTYLE

The mind is powerful in so many ways. It works its best when one begins to recognize that most of the things we see as bad in life are due to negative energy. We owe it to ourselves to live the best life possible and it starts with weeding out the negative energy surrounding our everyday existence. The negative energy can come from yourself; the people you surround yourself with; your daily activities that may include the programs you watch on TV, the music you listen to, the medication you take, foods you eat, etc.

Negativity in the mind can have you look at a positive situation in a negative manner. You need to focus on looking at things in a positive manner. As the saying goes, from all bad comes good, from trial and tribulations comes strength and so on. You need to begin to focus on turning everything around from negative to positive energy. Mind focus, as I love to call it, is your state of utilizing your mind to bring about the best positive energy; the energy that keeps

How I Do It

you focused on your mission.

     Having said all that, start your journey into a fitness lifestyle by using "mind focus" and choose the activities that you enjoy. You do not need to belong to a gym to be able to workout. You may do activities outside of a gym like riding a bike, rollerblading, roller-skating, running, dancing, etc. The fact is you have to keep the body in motion and if you choose something you enjoy, you will stick with it and eventually learn how to diversify your workouts as you fall in love with your fitness lifestyle.

How I Do It

Notes

Chapter Three

NUTRITION (SPORTS)

The RDA is a good reference for the average person. However, for an individual that partakes in more than the 30 minutes/3x a week workout, there are supplements and vitamins that can be taken according to your training plan. In addition, for individuals with ailments that are on prescribed medication or in need of additional nutrient support; a more extreme look into the dietary needs must be evaluated by a licensed practitioner.

I want to begin by pointing out that while I will explain my intake of nutrients below, I want you to recognize a general rule I use quite religiously. I allow my sugar intake to be **9 grams or less per each meal/snack.** This sugar intake will vary depending on what training I am doing or my physiological state. I average my food intake at approximately 1600 to 2000 calories per day. And, of course, it will definitely vary on when I have my cheat meal or indulge on vacation. In addition, I never allow my calories to go under my Basal Metabolic Rate (BMR) as that would cause a decline in the results of my training plan.

Furthermore, I cycle my carbohydrates based

How I Do It

on gaining mass or trimming down. What I do is add approximately 200 calories or so on the days that I am focusing on building mass. I then will choose a couple days within that week to reduce my carbohydrates intake by 200 calories or so. I do not measure or weigh my food as I have a pretty good idea of my portion sizes. In the past, I have used the palm of my hand to get a general idea of my protein intake. I basically use that method for everything except my fats. For trimming down, I basically reduce my sugar and carbohydrates intake by 200 calories or so for a few days. I often do not have to do this because I eat pretty clean most of the time.

Protein Intake

As for my protein nutrient, I make it a point to eat 5 to 6 mini meals a day. However, there are days that I eat more than that and more often than 2 1/2 hours apart. I digest approximately 25 grams of protein per each meal however, when I am eating more than my standard 5 to 6 mini meals, I do not include 25grams of protein after the 6th meal. Too much protein in the body has been debated by a number of organizations in causing bone or joint disorder problems like gout and osteoporosis due to uric acid buildup. There is no real proof of this but I try to keep my protein at bodyweight(**BW**) or my **BW** with an additional 25 to 50% of **BW** on my heavier training days where I feel that muscle recovery warrants this consumption. On lighter

How I Do It

training days, I stick with protein consumption ranging from 90% of **BW** to full **BW**.

The protein sources that I eat regularly are eggs (1 yolk for every 3 eggs), tilapia, pollock, salmon, tuna, sardines, chicken, black beans, spinach, protein shakes and protein bars.

Carbohydrates Intake

One important factor in **building muscle** is to make certain to continue eating complex carbohydrates. I increase my carbohydrates and find that the common food of choice is pizza. I will add tuna to it as it works very well for me. You need to EAT to grow!

Since I am in the perimenopausal state, I find that as my body stresses I begin to incorporate the "B" vitamins as well as eating more complex carbohydrates to sustain my much-needed energy levels. The carbohydrates that I include quite readily are black beans and high fiber tortilla wraps. You have to understand that if the body does not receive the nutrients it needs to balance your hormone levels; it begins to stress causing the body to cycle downward and energy levels to decline. In fact, take note that when your cortisol levels rise; they cause your body to hold onto unwanted fat.

How I Do It

Fruits and vegetables are extremely important in sustaining energy levels along with the repair of all building blocks in the body. Therefore, I make certain to eat plenty of fruits and vegetables; however, the quantity and timeframe may vary depending on my stress levels. I, for the most part, try to have my fruit intake early during the day and eliminate it altogether or minimize it from the afternoon on until bedtime as fruits contain a lot of sugar. I only alter this when my body tells me that I am lacking that nutrient in my body. Remember, always listen to your body-it will guide you in what you need unless you suffer certain ailments that may deter the senses from responding well.

Fat Intake

I consume good fats like almonds, walnuts, fish oils, flax oil (on occasion), regular/organic olive oil, peanuts, almond butter, soynut butter, avocado, regular/organic peanut butter, pistachios, all nuts. On various occasions, I may consume a product with coconut oil or a light cheese product to rev up the fat metabolism process. However, I rarely utilize the coconut oil as I keep my fat burning engine fueled by consuming my mini meals with some form of good fat. The aforementioned are sources of one of the following in the unsaturated family of fats - **Omega 3**(ALA-Alpha-linolenic Acid, EPA-Eicosapentaenoic Acid, DHA-Docosahexaenoic Acid, SDA-Stearidonic Acid), **Omega 6**(GLA-Gamma-linolenic Acid,

How I Do It

DGLA-Dihomogamma-linolenic Acid, LA-Linoleic Acid, AA-Arachidonic Acid), **Omega 7**(BA-Butyric Acid, PA-Palmitic Acid & SA-Stearic Acid) or **Omega 9**(OA-Oleic Acid).

The aforementioned fats are those that I include in my 5 to 6 mini meals throughout the day. However, depending on the physique that I am looking for along with the demands of my body, I may alter the consumption.

The bad fats that you do not want in your diet are trans, hydrogenated and rancid. These fats include food sources such as margarine, shortenings, processed foods, packaged foods, frozen foods, fried snack foods, commercially baked cookies, cakes, etc.

Physique Appearance

As far as all my meals go, I alter them according to the physique I want to have in a given timeframe. If I am looking for a **ripped physique**, I reduce my carbohydrates(e.g., beans, breads, fruit) from noon until bedtime and increase protein intake to approximately 150% of my **BW** at about 25grams per meal. However, I will keep consuming vegetables like spinach, broccoli, asparagus, celery and mustard greens with my lean protein and fat (e.g., fish oil, almonds, peanuts) for all my meals.

If I am looking for the **sexy/bikini physique**

How I Do It

look, I simply continue with my complex carbohydrates prior to the very last meal. That last meal may consist of a protein shake with a fish oil capsule or protein shake with handful of almonds. I also incorporate dark organic chocolate with a protein shake during midday for this sexy look. Its antioxidant powers are amazing and keep me vibrant and feeling sexy along with serving as an anti-inflammatory due to its bioflavonoid and flavanols. In fact, the cocoa itself in dark chocolate is a good source of the minerals iron, calcium, magnesium, sulphur, zinc, copper, potassium, and manganese; plus some of the B Vitamins.

Noted next you will find that the Glycemic Foods Index Chart will give you a general idea of the range in glycemic count for that particular food source. This information may vary slightly based on various research sources. Low glycemic foods cause small blood sugar rises that do not last long thus minimizing or eliminating the trigger to fat storage. However, high glycemic foods have a larger rise in blood sugar that last longer and trigger fat storage.

How I Do It

GLYCEMIC FOODS INDEX

LOW 1 - 40 MED 40 - 80 HIGH 80 - 120

BREADS	**BREAKFAST**
Rye bread 48 Pita bread, whole wheat 57 Croissant 67 Oat bran bread 68 Mixed Grain Bread 69 Oatmeal 70 Pumpernickel 71 Pita Bread, white 82 Hamburger bun 87 Melba Toast 100 Bagel, white 103 Kaiser rolls 104 Bread stuffing 106 Rice Cakes 110 Wheat bread, Wonderwhite 112 Wheat bread, gluten free 129 French baguette 136	Rice bran 27 Kellogg's All Bran Fruit 'n Oats 55 All-bran 60 Granola Bars, Quaker Chew 61 Oatmeal 70 Bran Buds 75 Special K 77 Oat Bran 78 Kellogg's Honey Smacks 78 Muesli 80 Kellogg's Mini-Wheats 81 Bran Chex 83 Kellogg's Just Right 84 Life 94 Cream of Wheat 99 Golden Grahams 102 Puffed Wheat 105 Cheerios 106 Corn Bran 107 Nutri-grain 94 Grapenuts 96 Shredded Wheat 99

How I Do It

LEGUMES	PASTA
Lentils 41 Kidney beans 42 Garbanzo beans 47 Pinto beans 55 Black-eyed beans 59 Pinto beans, canned 64 Soy beans 25 Black beans, canned 69 Kidney beans, canned 69	Spaghetti, protein enriched 38 Fettuccini 46 Macaroni 64 Linguine 65 Instant Noodles 67 Ravioli, meat filled 56 Spaghetti, white 59 Spirali 61 Capellini 64 Tortellini, cheese 71 Macaroni and Cheese 92 Gnocchi 95 Potato, mashed 100

VEGETABLES	DAIRY
Peas, green 38 Sweet corn 55 White Potato 56 Sweet Potato 54 Yams 71 Carrots 71 Potato, white, boiled 80 Beets 91 Potato, mashed 100 Rutabaga 103 Pumpkin 107 Potato 120 Parsnips 131	Yogurt, lowfat, plain 20 Milk Chocolate 34 Milk, full fat 39 Milk, skim 46 Yogurt, low-fat, fruit 47 Ice cream, low-fat 71 Ice cream 87 **CRACKERS** Jatz 79 Wheat Crackers 96 Stoned Wheat Thins 96 Water Crackers 102 Rice Cakes 110 Puffed Crispbread 116

How I Do It

FRUITS Cherries 32 Grapefruit 36 Apple 38 Apple juice, unsweetened 40 Apricots, dried 44 Pear, fresh 53 Apple 54 Plum 55 Apple juice 58 Peach, fresh 60 Orange 53 Pear, canned 63 Grapes 66	Pineapple juice 66 Peach, canned 67 Grapefruit juice 69 Orange juice 74 Kiwi 75 Banana 77 Fruit cocktail 79 Mango 80 Apricots, fresh 82 Raisins 91 Apricots, canned syrup 91 Pineapple 94 Canteloupe) 93 Watermelon 103
SNACK FOODS Peanuts 21 Jams and marmalades 70 Skittles 98 Life Saver 100 Corn chips 105 Jelly Beans 114 Pretzels 116 Dates 146 Chocolate 70 Potato crisps 77 Popcorn 79	**SUGARS** Agave nectar 11 Fructose 32 Lactose 65 Honey 83 High fructose corn syrup 89 Sucrose 92 Glucose 137 **SOUPS** Tomato 54 Lentil canned 63 Split pea 89 Black bean 92 Green peas, canned 94

How I Do It

Notes

How I Do It

Chapter Four

SUPPLEMENTS

I take a daily multi-vitamin with my very first meal irrespective of what time it is in the day. Throughout the day I supplement with fish oils, B-Complex, Ester Vitamin C (easier on stomach) and Calcium. And sometimes when I need that extra kick or my body's hormones are off, I supplement with either B-complex or B6 and B12. I try not to use flaxseed unless I am constipated, due to high protein diet; as flaxseed minimizes the estrogen levels by bringing estrogen and progesterone at balance levels in a woman's body. As I am in my perimenopausal years, I need to keep all the estrogen possible to stay looking vibrant and minimize any stress associated with my menstrual cycle. Although the usage of flaxseed may prove otherwise for women with more fat on their bodies; I find it to be something that I would minimize or eliminate altogether. In addition, I alternate the use of soy products like soy milk, soy butter and organic soy yogurt to help increase my estrogen levels during this timeframe. I then immediately stop all soy products while on my menstruation and start up again a week prior to when my menstruation should begin.

How I Do It

I use whey and soy protein powders in a form of a shake. My shakes vary as I have quite a number of different concoctions that are listed in the Foods Chapter. I try to drink a protein shake with carbohydrates 30 to 45 minutes before working out. I will vary whether I take a fish oil capsule during this time as I may be focusing on burning the fat currently on my body. If not, I will add a fish oil capsule to my shake to have all nutrients flowing into my body in a normal pace as fat slows the digestion process and minimizes any high glycemic effect.

After my hard muscle-building workouts, I will drink a high-glycemic protein shake without any fish oil or any other type of fat. This allows the protein to flow much quicker into the bloodstream and feed the muscles to a faster recovery. In some cases, where I may not have exhausted my muscles to failure; I keep my post workout shake to low glycemic due to less needed muscle recovery.

As of date, I have never used fat burners or any energy fueled drinks. I use my Vitamin C and B vitamins to give me my fuel in addition to the foods I eat.

However, I want to point out that irrespective of where you are in your stage of life, ADLs and fitness journey; eating foods is far superior to supplements. Remember, supplements are just that-

How I Do It

supplements added to your food intake to meet the needs of your body's physical demands.

How I Do It

Notes

How I Do It

Chapter Five

STRETCHING AND WARMING UP

Stretching is very important especially when you transition your workout to muscle areas that are not trained on a regular basis. The lactic acid build up will cause soreness and sometimes can be very painful. Therefore, what I generally do is walk up and down my stairs several times and/or walk on the treadmill or wherever for 15 minutes in order to circulate the blood in my body and then I perform my stretches. You never want to stretch a cold muscle/joint. At post workout, you want to stretch again for another 15 minutes or more if the muscles you have trained are not regularly exercised. However, your body may still result in some soreness in those affected areas. I believe that instead of resting the next day, do a light workout by walking and moving the areas that are sore. You want blood circulation to occur so that the lactic acid is removed from the muscles.

In addition to this, what I **incorporate in my strength and/or resistance training is stretching in between my sets.** I find that this minimizes or eliminates any post soreness and helps with blood flow to those muscle fibers. I also make certain that

How I Do It

on any given day, I stretch my back in order to keep my back more flexible and minimize any tightening effect thus causing pressure on my discs. This is something I just do religiously with having bulging discs. Any form of sitting, standing; lying down, biking; etc. will use the back so keeping it flexible is one of my most important exercises.

Another method I use regularly is dancing to warm me up and then I stretch and continue onto my weight-training.

Lastly, I will choose one day per week where I do full-body stretches for approximately 1 hour. I stretch all parts of body (e.g., legs, arms, back, glutes, neck, abdominals, obliques). The stretching is done progressively where you reach and hold for 30 seconds and continue further into the stretch and repeat the hold for 30 seconds and so on. Once your muscle starts shaking-you have gone too far(clear sign for injury). At that point, gently release and back up to last stretch point. These full body stretch days are very invigorating as they relieve tension from all muscles and allow the release of toxins. After this full hour of stretch, try and drink plenty of water in order to get the maximum benefit of releasing those toxins.

How I Do It

Notes

How I Do It

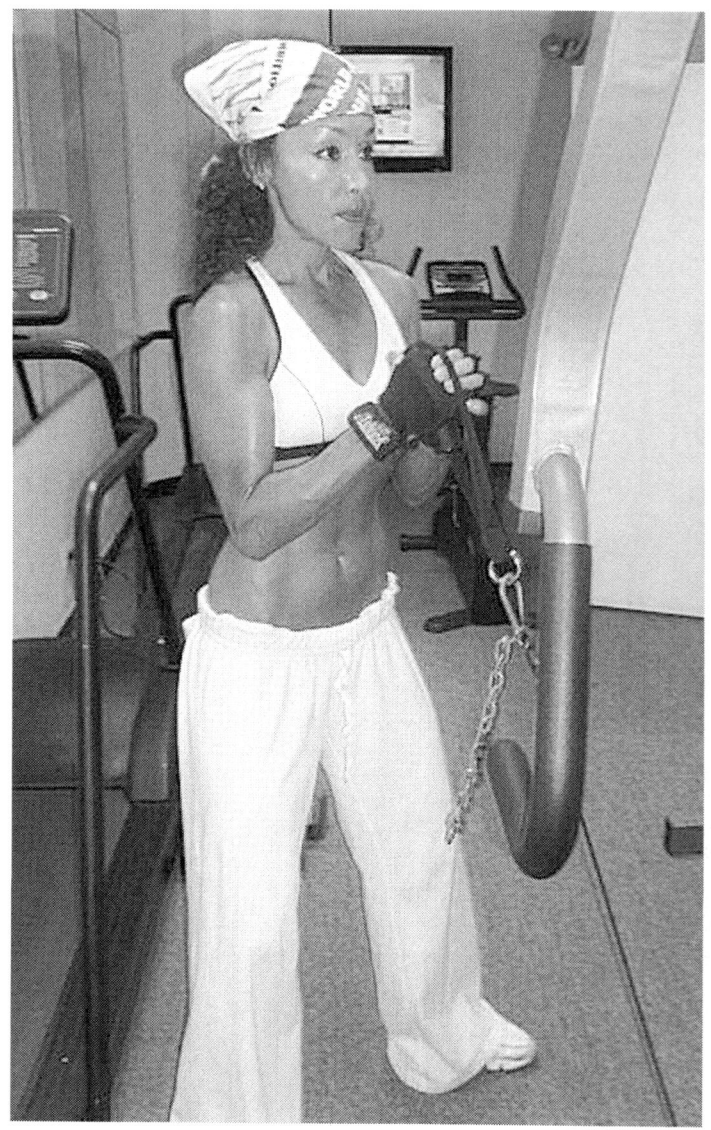

How I Do It

Chapter Six

STRENGTH TRAINING

For all my life, I have always been a very diversified woman. I have recognized that standard classes whether they be some type of aerobics class or any other type; I have never enjoyed the all in one fitness motto that serves for everyone. I have always enjoyed doing my own workout routines, dancing, dressing with a difference twist; just always being more of a leader than a follower.

Therefore, I have developed these routines as they not only provide more of a well-rounded infused muscular contraction but incorporate cardiovascular exercise within them to continue building those feel good endorphins. These feel good endorphins provide pain and soreness relief during and after my workouts. With this type of training, I am getting the benefits of strength and cardiovascular all in one. Take note that depending on your physiological state, certain training methods may or may not work well for you but understand that I am explaining my methods of training to stay fit and as youthful as possible throughout my current stage of life.

I have set out some of the various workouts I

perform broken up by abdominals, obliques, lower and upper body; and back/chest resistance training. This training provides muscular contraction to the noted areas in various different methods. I use all these methods and vary them according to my stress levels, time-constraints, location and/or perimenopausal symptoms.

ABDOMINAL EXERCISES

Through my decades of exercise; I have found the importance and benefits of using proper midsection form. This usage allows you to get an automatic abs workout with every exercise movement you perform. Remember, the midsection (abdominals and oblique) are muscles just like any others that need rest. In fact, when you really think about it; they are being used all the time if you use proper midsection form. Therefore, you may find that overworking these muscles may not give you the totally toned or ripped abdominals effect.

Furthermore, you will find that since I use proper midsection form for all my training; I am able to develop and sculpt the body while preventing injuries. I only have to do a couple abdominal and oblique exercises once a month. I have no more need for midsection training if my nutrition plan is intact and proper midsection form technique is performed during every exercise.

How I Do It

Note: These following individual exercises are in a repetition of only 3 sets.

(1) I perform the hanging leg raises with knees slightly bent raising them up to pelvic level repeatedly until failure.

(2) In order to prevent any back pain or pressure on my bulging discs, I lay on the floor in supine position (with back to floor); lift both legs with slightly bent knees and bring as high up until I feel the burn in my abdominals. I repeat this until failure. I then do my second set at **50% of the raise** and then hold legs in upward position until failure.

Please Note: Exercise 2 works the Abdominals without adding pressure to my back and hips as it is more stable then the pull on the back in the hanging leg raise. That is why I do the hanging leg raise maybe once every 2 months.

Also, I never add leg weights to do the abdominal exercises as that will only cause more pressure to the back and create more unnecessary stress.
There is no need to add weights to this exercise to get amazing abs. It is not about the weight, it is about the infused pressure of the contraction of that muscle.

(3) Lay supine and bring legs upward with knees slightly bent (less stress on lower back); continue to

How I Do It

breathe in and out alternating by **spreading legs outward** and bring legs upwards with knees still slightly bent. This outward leg upward swing exercise works the abs but focuses **more concentration on the front oblique areas.** In addition to the aforementioned movements, you can include a 5lb. dumbbell and lift your upper body while holding the weight over chest area with arms spread reaching towards ceiling. This extra move will definitely have upper and lower abdominals working to their max potential. You can increase the dumbbell weight, as you feel comfortable with the results of your training. Perform until failure.

(4) Get into push up position for the abdominal plank. This is one of my favorites as it works the shoulders, chest and abdominals along with back. Bring your right arm to elbow bend resting on floor while left arm is in full stretch/extension. Then, alternate the movement bending left arm to elbow and extending right arm. Perform until failure. The movements here are working those aforementioned muscles at different ranges and providing cardiovascular activity with this power exercise.

OBLIQUE EXERCISES
Note: The following individual exercises are in a repetition of only 3 sets.

(1) Lay on either side in plank position and lower

How I Do It

your waist towards floor without touching it; then bring it back up-do as many as you can with your own bodyweight. If you want to increase the burn/intensity, add a weight ball to this exercise. Hold onto the ball centering it to your abdominal area with the hand that is not used to hold you in plank position and continue same exercise. Switch sides and do same format. Perform until failure.

(2) I use a bosu ball, lay my back on it as if I were going to do crunches and I sometimes hold a weight ball or weight in center of abs and rotate my upper body to the right and then rotate to the left. **I do as many until failure.** This method of exercise gives you the burn that you are looking for to develop some nicely sculpted obliques. And, of course, you can do this exercise without any added weight ball or weight but your own bodyweight. **My preference is with bodyweight only to prevent any further pressure on my back.** Perform until failure.

(3) I also perform hanging oblique leg raises where I actually hold onto the bar with my arms extended and I bring my right hip area up into an inward rotation towards the left side and do the opposite movement with my left hip side. Perform until failure.

(4) Another hanging oblique leg raise exercise is that instead of doing rotation, you bring your legs straight up slowing **but spreading them apart as far as you**

How I Do It

can go with slight bent of the knees to eliminate any back/hip pressure. Do this until failure. It is tougher than the normal abs leg raises where both legs come up in closed position. Perform until failure.

I do not perform very many exercises in the way of a weight rotation position that directly concentrate on the obliques. The reason for this is that due to my bulging discs, the weight pressure would just cause my discs to bulge further. I obviously have found safer methods to keep my obliques in tiptop shape.

In the past, I have used other exercises with a cable pulley. You stand sideways pulling the cable and bend sideways. However, I have found that this repetitive motion can actually over time; aggravate the lower back discs and I would not suggest it. Furthermore, this direct movement of bending sideways builds the obliques outward instead of slimming inward for the more desirable v-shape look.

LOWER BODY WORKOUTS

All the exercise routines I have designed through improvisation with the notion of less stress while infusing the various muscle groups. I do them all to failure with adjusting the weight based on my stress and/or physiological state.

How I Do It

I would suggest that you most certainly do a 12-count repetition of that particular exercise being discussed before hitting your failure point. However, if you reach failure before 12 reps; lighten up on the weight until you can do at least 12 repetitions.

In addition, I want to point out that muscle fibers play a big role in your development of muscle tissue/mass. For me, I have found that lighter weights with more repetition work best as I apparently have Type I muscle fibers. The opposite is true for people with Type II muscle fibers.

Note: All the following exercises in these routines can be done as individual exercises according to your fitness level.

Exercise Routine One - Glutes and Legs

Step 1. Lunges - Perform lunge by simply using your bodyweight and stay in position **for 5 to 10 seconds** while stretching into the lunge. This is more of a pilates-infused type position. Step forward into your lunge and bend knee not passing toes and alternate knee should not touch floor; you will feel the burn in the quadriceps, hamstrings and gluteal areas. The lunge can be done with continuous forward walking or in one position stepping forward into your lunge position and then back. You do not need to have a lot a space to accomplish this exercise. Perform as

How I Do It

many to failure.
Then walk for a few minutes;
Step 2. <u>Bunny Hop Mountain Climbers</u> - Get into a push-up position and fully extend both of your legs. Then use both legs to jump into chest position and back to extended leg position. **I call these bunny hops.** Perform as many to failure.
Then jog for a few minutes;
Step 3. Speed rope for 30 seconds or 1 minute. If you do not have a speed rope then improvise and jump in standalone position.
Repeat Routine One 3 to 5 Times

These methods of Pilate-Yoga infused workouts provide the muscle to be under tension longer durations. While the weight load may not contain any additional weight other than your own, the exertion that the muscle will be under is the resistance of pressure. To me, these are some of the most stress-free workouts because they have no added weight and therefore any back pressure can be minimized or eliminated altogether. Now remember proper form is key. If you feel pain-STOP! You may have gone too far into the stretch and caution is advised in order to prevent any injury. Remember, a good burning sensation primarily lets you know that you have that muscle under resistance. However, if you experience pain, that is not a good sign. The saying "no pain no gain" was not telling you to go to the extent of a painful situation. It referred to the burning sensation you should feel that indicates the muscle is under resistance and the muscle fibers are activated at that time.

Exercise Routine Two - Glutes

Step 1. Walk on treadmill for 30 minutes at lower cardiovascular rate for your age.
Then
Step 2. Glute Kickups - With or without ankle weights on legs, get into kneeling position with hands down and do kickups by extending your right leg back and continuing the push upward effect without returning to start position, do as many and hold last repetition to failure; repeat same exercise with left leg;
Then walk/stretch for a couple minutes;
Step 3. Sidekicks - In standing position, perform sidekicks working those abductor muscles in the hip/thigh area. Swing your leg outward to the side as far high as you can go and perform reps until failure. Alternate leg and do same format. (**Note: I will include inward kicks once a month using my adductor muscles as I find that with all my workouts I keep them strong enough**)
Then walk for a couple minutes;
Step 4. Perform lunges as noted in **Exercise Routine One**;
Then walk for a couple minutes;
Step 5. Infused Squat - Get into a squat-infused position - (get into squat position lowering body into

a sitting position keeping knees from passing your toes and spreading arms forward for balance. Hold position until failure while **pressing down on your heels lifting toes slightly**-this gives that extra burn to the gluteal area.
Then walk/stretch for a couple minutes;
Step 6. Stretch out your lower body; particularly your sides as the midsection has definitely been used for proper form stability in this mode of infused muscular diversification exercise;
Repeat Routine Two 3 to 5 times
Then and finally;
Step 7. Dance 10 minutes or so to whatever music you enjoy preferably in warm room for max burn of calories! (Sweat them toxins right out of your body). The dance movements that shake your butt continue the flow of blood into the worked out muscle areas **(continues feeding muscle fibers with necessary nutrients if you properly supplemented and didn't overtrain).**

How I Do It

Exercise Routine Three - Legs and Glutes

Step 1. Do 20 minutes of walking on treadmill; **start incline at level 4 and continually increase (according to your fitness level) and only perform at fat burn rate.** You are starting your weight training right on the treadmill as you feel your legs and glutes contract due to the slower walk and continually incline.
Then
Step 2. Quadriceps - Use the leg extension machine that concentrates on the quadriceps for 5 sets for a count of 12 to 20. Try to go as heavy as possible and hit the 20th repetition. If stress levels are high, do lighter weights until failure. On these days, I will go usually as high as 35 repetitions with lighter weights.
Then stretch quads;
Then
Step 3. Hamstrings - Use the seated leg curl machine that concentrates on the hamstrings. Repeat same format as **Step 2. Quadriceps.**
Then stretch hams;
Then
Step 4. All - Use the leg press machine for working the calves, quads, hamstrings and glutes. **I will reposition the chair closer for each set, totaling 5 sets of a 20 repetition count**. By repositioning, you are hitting different areas of the muscle thus giving that entire muscle a more infused burn. The gluteal area is hit more intensely by repositioning and pushing

ONLY with the heel of your foot-a method I use to infuse those muscles. For my bulging discs, I will place my hands on my lower back for more stability.
Then
Step 5. I will walk 20 minutes after workout. However, the walking varies based on what nutrition plan I am on and other physiological factors. For example, I will opt. to do this if I am focusing on burning fat and will perform cardio only at fat level.
Repeat Routine Three 3 to 5 times

NOTE: I incorporate or replace Step 3 with the gluteal/hamstring machine. In addition, I will allow my legs to hang down on this machine and bring both legs up in backward movement to develop and strengthen the glutes. *I will keep my legs up and rotate my legs in a small circular movement while pushing upwards and sideways to infuse the entire gluteal muscles.*

Exercise Routine Four - Glutes

Step 1. Use leg press machine with open ends to both sides of it. **(How I use it with bulging discs).** In my experience, I have found that if I want to increase the weight load to the traditional leg press machine I would rather improvise it with this machine due to possibly aggravating my back and further pushing out my discs. Therefore this is how I have improvised the

How I Do It

usage of the leg press machine that has openings to both sides of it, right and left. These machines are typically found in small gyms, apartment building gyms, etc.

I will stand on the left side of machine leaning part of my right side of body in straight/vertical position. I then will hold firmly onto back of seat and position my right leg **with foot tilted slightly right and heel pressing down on press**, select my weight amount based on 25 to 30 reps and perform 3 to 5 sets. Thereafter, I switch sides and continue same format with left side. Now, remember you can alternate between sets from one side to another.
Then
Step 2. I perform 3 minutes or less of jumping in place (speed rope if available).
Then
Step 3. <u>Do step forward plies</u>. I will do this dance move in a slow pace bringing right foot forward with outward tilt pressing into toe area to get **gluteal and calf areas to burn**. By stepping into this position and holding for 10 seconds or more, you will be infusing those muscles giving you more of a strength and toning workout. Repeat this until failure. Repeat with left foot and do same format.
Note: You can increase your cardiovascular workout by doing these plies in jumping forward format instead of slow movement. I alternate and do this move every other repetition of routine.

How I Do It

Repeat Routine Four 3 to 5 times

Exercise Routine Five - Calves and Shoulders (upper body included)

Note: Warm-up for 15 mins. with any type of cardio.

Step 1. <u>Calves</u> - (Improvisation that works the calves and lower hamstring harder-my favorite) if gym does not have appropriate calf machine to work this muscle, use the seated leg extension machine for quads by standing facing front of machine. Then position both legs in back of roller, lock your hands and arms in a comfortable position holding on to the front of this machine or the seat-whatever feels comfortable to you. Then begin by pushing back with one leg/ankle at a time. I find that using this machine works my calves and lower hamstrings a lot harder than using the leg press or leg extension machines for this exercise. **I have improvised my calf and hamstring training with this machine as I have found it to provide much more definition to the upper part of my calves and lower hamstrings. Then stretch calves and hams;**
Then
Step 2. Calf Bounces - Simply stand (holding onto wall for support or place hands on waist) and lift your body up by pressing on toes and lifting heels in bouncing effect; continue until failure;
Then walk/stretch calves;

Then
Step 3. <u>Shoulders Military Press</u> - Perform military press raises with two dumbbells. You can do this seated or standing; whatever feels more comfortable to you. Start with the dumbbells in your hands and raise your arms so that your hands are on opposite sides of your head, elbows bent and in line with your shoulders. Bring them overhead but do not have dumbbells touch and keep a slight bent in elbows. **Do not lock the joint.**
Then Repeat Step 1.;
Then
Step 3. <u>Shoulders Front Raise</u>- Perform a shoulder front raise with what I call infusing the anterior deltoids. Do it standing or sitting but remember to use your midsection to keep you stable. Bring both arms forward in front of your body with dumbbells in hand; return to start position, ***but continually shift your arms outward by a few inches as you continue the lifting forward position***. Once you have repeated exercise to finally a lateral raise, (arms extended to the side) return to starting the front raise and so on until you have at least reached 12 repetitions or until failure. **NOTE: Three times a month I take my raises a bit past the center level of the shoulders. I push my arms slightly back to hit my posterior deltoids. I will also do reverse flyes during this time.**

Repeat Routine Five 3 to 5 times

Exercise Routine Six- Legs and Glutes (Drop Sets)

Note: I perform this particular workout on my non-stressful days as this workout requires some heavy duty exertion. I love drops sets because they really shock the body with heavy intensity training. *Also, to diversify this workout routine; try moving your leg alignment on equipment a bit for every set to get a full muscle workout.

Note: Warm-up for 15 mins. with any type of cardio.

Step 1. Quadriceps - Use the quadriceps leg extension machine. Make certain that your amount of weight is enough for 10 repetitions in 1 set. After performing the 10 repetitions, simply drop the weight by 5 lbs. and within 10 to 15 seconds-continue with next set of 10 repetitions. Continue with weight drops and do a maximum of 5 drop sets of 10 reps each.

Then stretch quads/walk for a few minutes;

Step 2. Hamstrings - Use the hamstring curl machine (anyone) and perform exact method as in **Step 1**.

Then stretch hams/walk for a few minutes;

Step 3. Glutes - Use butt buster machine or similar one with the ability to push your legs, one at a time, backwards and upward. Perform same drop method with this machine as in **Step 1**. *Note: You will find that the hamstrings and calves are getting hit as well.*

Then walk for a minute in long lunge leg format

How I Do It

stretches.
Repeat Routine Six 3 to 5 times

How I Do It

UPPER BODY WORKOUTS

Exercise Routine One - Refer to Exercise Routine Five from Lower Body Workouts as it includes two exercises for shoulders.
Repeat Routine One 3 to 5 times

Exercise Routine Two - Shoulders, Biceps & Triceps

Note: Warm-up for 15 mins. with any type of cardio.
Step 1. All - Grab a pair of dumbbells or resistance band and start doing **boxing movements**. You can increase the muscle tension by slowing the movement process (**start with a count of 4 and gradually increase to 10 as your fitness level deems**) and feeling the burn as you take the muscle into the concentric and eccentric moves. By doing so, you are activating muscle fibers through this slight boxing rotation. After doing 20 - 30 reps, stretch the affected area;
Then dance for a minute or so;
Step 2. Shoulders Military Press - With equipment in **Step 1**, perform your shoulder overhead raise and **slow the motion** for more activated muscle contraction. (**In Exercise Routine Five Step. 3**)
Then dance for a minute or so;
Step 3. Incline Biceps Curls/Shoulders Front Raise

How I Do It

- With equipment in **Step 1** and a bench or whatever you find suitable to recline in and stable your body. (**I use my bed at times**). Perform your biceps curls by positioning your body at an incline of 90-degree angle and **slowly** bring the weight to your front deltoid. **(Into half of your reach-rotate weight outward to get a more infused burn on the anterior deltoid).** Do as many and hold last repetition to failure.
*Also, take note that you can slightly rotate the weights in an outward position during your lifting movement thereby hitting the various areas of those muscles.
Then dance for a minute or so;
Step 4. <u>Incline Triceps Kickback</u> - With equipment in **Step 1**, bend forward about 90 degrees and perform your triceps extensions(kickbacks) swinging your arms **slowly** backwards without locking the joint. Do as many and hold last repetition to failure.
Repeat Routine Two 3 to 5 times

Note: These workouts are especially good during those stressful periods where lifting heavy will just put you in an overstressed state thus promoting fat storage. Also, be aware that the more you manipulate the incline in your exercises, you get a more distributed resistance on the muscle thus overall strength balance.

How I Do It

Exercise Routine Three - Biceps & Back Infused

Note: Warm-up for 15 mins. with any type of cardio.
Step 1. Biceps Angled Curls - Grab a pair of dumbbells and a bench with incline. Incline to your desire and begin your bicep curls by bringing dumbbells up *slightly rotating the dumbbell right during your lifting movement.* This will make the biceps pop and give you a more balanced bicep muscle. Do as many and hold last repetition to failure.
Then walk a minute or so;
Step 2. Bent-over Dumbbell Row - With dumbbells in hands, bend over with back being parallel to floor. Bring arms up towards back together bending at elbows. Do not bypass your back. Do as many and hold last repetition to failure.
Then walk a minute or so;
Step 3. Biceps Curls - In standing position, bring dumbbells upward to mid-level at abs location. Do as many and hold last repetition to failure.
Then walk a minute or so;
Step 4. Lower Back Pulls - In standing position, adjust wide bar or double-handle rope on cable pulley. Step back pulling on pulley towards back bringing elbows in bent position. Do not bypass your back. Do as many and hold last repetition to failure.
Repeat Routine Three 3 times

How I Do It

Exercise Routine Four - Shoulders
This routine I do with dumbbells as well. However, the reason why I switch to a *circular weight* is for the *weight distribution it offers*. I find that rotating these workouts keeps shocking my body to create a more balanced shoulder muscle structure.

Note: Warm-up for 15 mins. with any type of cardio.
Step 1. Shoulder Front/Middle Raise - In either sitting or standing position, grab a circular weight from the rack (5lb weight or less/more depending on your strength level) placing fingers through middle hole of weights and bring them upward with arms wide open *above and slightly forward* from shoulder level. You should be feeling a contraction burn on the front/middle(outer) deltoids. Do as many repetitions to failure but not less than 12.
Then walk a minute or so;
Step 2. Side Laydown Shoulder Raise - Get a bench or bosu ball and position yourself **lying sideways** with **your upper body elevated by 90 degrees**. Bend your arm very slightly at elbow, bring it up sideways to almost shoulder length and feel the contraction/burn in your middle/outer deltoid area with part of bicep/tricep areas being hit. Do as many to failure but not less than 12. Switch sides and repeat with other arm.
Then walk a minute or so;
Step 3. Shoulder Lateral Raise - In standing

How I Do It

position, hold the circular weight and bring your arm directly out to the side leveling at almost shoulder. You should feel a burn in the middle(outer) deltoid area. **You can do both arms at a time or single arm for a more infused contraction.**
Repeat Routine Four 3 to 5 times

BACK/CHEST WORKOUTS

Note: I want to point out that I do incorporate the traditional staples of working out the back and biceps, chest and triceps, shoulder with calves, etc. I will also do the push/pull methods. Any of the aforementioned I only perform once a month. I prefer diversifying my workouts as they seem to work very well for me.

Exercise Routine One

Note: Warm-up for 15 mins. with any type of cardio.
Step 1. Back Angled Pulldowns - Grab the double-handle rope and attach to cable pulley. Stand in front of pulley while bending forward-approx. 90 degrees. Pull the rope downward in angled position towards shoulders for your lats to feel the contraction. Do as many and hold last repetition to failure.
Then walk a minute or so;
Step 2. Incline Chest Press - Use a bench with

incline on it. Position the incline at a comfortable level. Grab a pair of dumbbells and bring both arms together over chest and towards ceiling, repeat until failure; *Note: During my sets, I diversify by the way the palm of your hand is facing when bringing dumbbells together-palms can face toward you, face each other or face away-I do all.*
Then walk a minute or so;
Step 3. <u>Back Pulldown</u> - Grab flat wide bar and attach to cable pulley. Stand straight in front of pulley and pull down to shoulder level feeling the contraction on the back of deltoids and lats. Do as many and hold last repetition to failure.
Then walk a minute or so;
Step 4. Repeat Step(**2**) but incline the bench further upward or downward in order to get a different range of muscle contraction in the chest area.
Repeat Routine One 3 times

Exercise Routine Two

Note: Warm-up for 15 mins. with any type of cardio.
Step 1. <u>Back Long Cable Pulls</u> - Grab bench and situate it in front of cable pulley. Use either double-pull rope or wide bar on pulley. Sit (**erect with abs in tight**) on the bench facing pulley and grab bar/rope and go as far back on bench as you can go. Pull on rope/bar inward towards chest area. Do as many and hold last repetition to failure.

How I Do It

Then walk a minute or so;
Step 2. <u>Chest</u> - Perform as many push-ups on floor until failure;
Then walk a minute or so;
Step 3. <u>Back One Arm Bent Rows</u> - Use bench situated in front of pulley equipment from **Step (1) above**. Grab a dumbbell, lean your body on bench with left knee, use left arm to hold firmly on bench while extending the right leg. With elbow bent, bring the right arm with dumbbell upward towards back but not bypassing your back. Do as many and hold last repetition to failure.
Then walk a minute or so;
Step 4. <u>Incline Chest Pushups</u> - Use bench situated in front of pulley equipment from **(Step 1)** and perform push-ups in an upward incline angle. Your hands should be placed on side edge of bench for stability and legs extended.
Repeat Routine Two 3 times
Please Note: Push-ups can be done with full legs extended or knees bent. Perform according to your fitness level.

I want to conclude this section in saying that if you have a particular area/muscle that has been injured and you cannot work that area by doing repetitions of really any amount of weight. Then take into consideration stabilizing movements.

For example, the side plank for obliques

How I Do It

works my obliques to the maximum. I do not ever have to worry about adding a weight-ball to that exercise. If my lower back is bothering me, I simply will hold the position for resistance until failure. Therefore, I do not have to further aggravate my lower back discs. So consider the injured muscle and perform a 1-repetition exercise without any weights. Hold that position until failure. You will be surprised how much you can develop and tone a muscle just by doing this infused muscle exercise. I started using this method after my back injury in 2007 as I did not want to use any weight training rotation machines or any other type of weighted equipment that would aggravate my back discs.

How I Do It

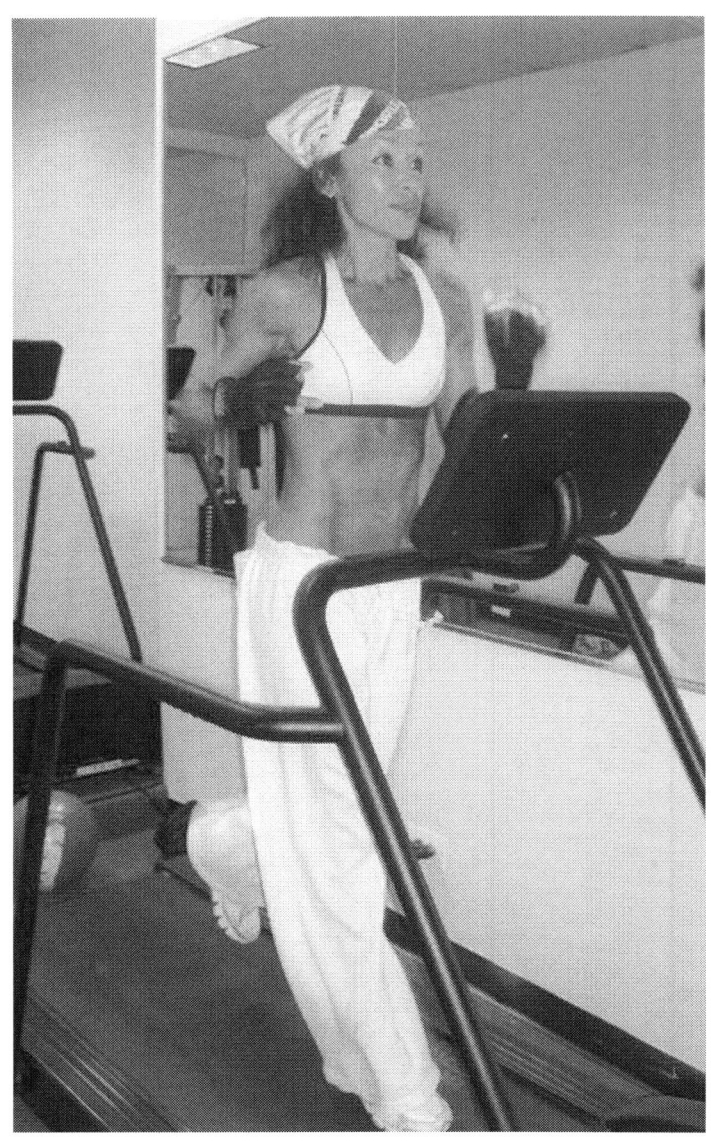

How I Do It

Chapter Seven

CARDIOVASCULAR EXERCISE

In some of my workouts, I will interject spontaneous running on a treadmill between my sets of weight training. This type of interval training is shocking the body in small spurts thus allowing less stress on my body as well as keeping it more toned by not causing atrophy to the muscles used with cardiovascular overtraining. This is as much running that I will do as I am on hiatus from running long distance.

I also incorporate the rowing machine. I use this machine for the cardio benefits but I interject some diversification with the arm/hand movement. While working out on this machine, I will perform the standard row movement with hand palms facing down on grips that work the triceps as well as the back. However, after about 50 repetitions of that movement, I will switch the hand palms facing upward to do my row movement thus working the biceps. I will continue for approximately 20 to 45 minutes rotating these movements based on reps and on how much cardio I feel I need to do that particular day.

How I Do It

Jumping rope is another form of beneficial cardiovascular workout that I perform when I interject this into my training plan. You can also improvise by just jumping in place or doing jumping jacks. When I do perform this exercise I simply do it for a few minutes or less and then continue with whatever other exercises are in my training plan. I also sometimes jump in standalone position allowing my mind to take me elsewhere. I have managed to do this for 1 hour in a small confined room during my 20s.

I also include **forward/backward jumping** with both legs and alternate with one leg at a time as this works the entire leg muscles along with the glutes. If you stabilize your position, your abs are working at the same time. **You can diversify this method of jumping by simply rotating your foot outwardly and pressing on toes when you jump that leg forward and you will contract the calf and glute muscle in a different angle.** Also diversify the jump by **crossing your legs** during the movement of the jump. You will feel the thighs working a bit harder.

Biking is another cardiovascular workout that I will try to perform once a week but find myself doing it more during summer months due to taking advantage of the beautiful weather and the healing powers from the Sun.

How I Do It

My stair stepping is done on various machines(e.g., stairmaster, glider) to angle the glutes and legs at various positions. This provides the means of overall contraction to those muscles thus allowing far more balanced muscular strength to those areas. When performing this exercise, always use proper form by keeping yourself erect and holding abs in tight-DON'T SLOUCH.

I perform mountain climbers as a cardiovascular workout to get my heart rate up and blasting fat while working the legs and glutes. I will **jump both legs (Bunny Hoppers)** in and out and alternate with single legs.

During winter when driving caution is advised, I will walk and/or run up and down my stairs depending on my stress levels. I walk regularly up and down my stairs throughout the day so incorporating this to my daily fitness lifestyle is quite feasible. Sometimes, I will opt to include some dumbbells to get that heart rate going a bit sooner along with getting some strength training in the arms. I will perform biceps and shoulder workouts while going up and down my stairs-**obviously I am walking carefully up and down when incorporating weights into the mix.**

Last, but certainly not least, I love to use

How I Do It

dancing as a form of cardiovascular and bodyweight workout. I use upbeat dance music that allows me to work my entire body especially my abdominals and obliques. I do hip thrust and rotation movements when dancing to give my core some training and keep my midsection looking great. I also incorporate stepping into back plies to work the gluteal muscles. It is truly amazing how much of a workout this is without any added weights thus eliminating additional stress. In addition, I use very light weights about 2 1/2 to 5 lbs and use them during my arm dance movements. It is amazing how toned and defined your arms can get with the usage of very little weight with much repetition.

How I Do It

Notes

How I Do It

Chapter Eight

CONTROLLING STRESS

Allergies were something foreign to me until I hit the age of 45. I have found that certain pollen during the summer, whether locally or not, would cause a headache, chest to tighten; and congestion would appear causing difficulty in breathing. For me, I take over-the-counter medication to put my allergies at bay in order for me to perform the basic ADLs along with my training. These are just signs that the body begins to lose certain hormones that are utilized as anti-inflammatory agents in the body. It is important to understand how this works in relative to the stress imposed on our body so that we properly supplement and medicate according to our needs. It is situations like these that I have found so many women decide to forget about starting and/or continuing their fitness journey. I understand my body more and its needs and therefore I am able to take the necessary care to continue my journey in a more positive and healthy manner.

During this time, I perform infused workouts by stretching and holding the muscle contractions for a minimum of 30 seconds. Try to resist from doing any stressful cardiovascular or weight-training

How I Do It

activities as well as eliminating any other stressful situations.

During these stressful times of perimenopause, the estrogen is low and the body will stress more in order to create the menstruation. I have begun to eat more soy-based products as they help in creating the estrogen I need. I also eliminated flaxseed from my diet in order to prevent the reduction of estrogen in my body. I continue my other supplements that include fish oil, vitamins B6, B12 and C.

Furthermore, some physicians recommend that sex is a great way to reduce stress. If you have no partner, masturbation is another form to create estrogen. I bet a lot of you did not know that masturbation actually helps in the process of creating estrogen.

Also, since this time brings about more vanity issues for most women, feel free to meditate and pray about your needs. Go out and get a manicure, pedicure and/or facial to feel better. Soak in a hot tub. Put on make-up, go out dancing, and put something sexy on. Do something that helps bring that sexy alive.

How I Do It

Notes

Chapter Nine

OVERCOMING AN INJURY

Since I have been involved in some form of fitness since the prime age of 12, I certainly have had my share of injuries. I pulled both hamstrings quite a few times and suffered a tendon tear in the groin area. The tendon tear in the groin area was at the age of 27 where I was at my peak of running. Some of the other injuries I sustained were pulled muscles in back, shoulder blades that recovered within a week or so. Some of these injuries might have been due to overtraining, not warming up and stretching improperly. However, the biggest and most traumatic injury I suffered was the herniation of my discs L4, L5 and S1 back in 2007 and then again 2008. My belief is that this traumatic injury was due to the gradual process of time as an athlete. As a matter a fact, I did not ever suffer from any back pain until January 2007 at the age of 43 upon the herniation of these discs.

However, because my endorphins were so high, I did not feel the pain at its worst as my sports physician had confirmed that notion. However, I was led to believe by my sports doctor that in six months I could increase my training with weights and running

How I Do It

all to find out that it was not the case. I relapsed and suffered another disc herniation six months later.

I decided to take my health into my own hands. I listened to my body and did not consult any further with my physicians other than to take medications for pain and anxiety caused by the sustained injuries.

I went on to lay off my training for an entire month, which seemed like a year to me. I did very little walking and continued to perform my stretching as my body continued to heal. I took my supplements: fish oil, B-Complex, B12, calcium and glucosamine for approximately six months. After my one-month hiatus from training, I decided to start back slowing with light weights and eliminate any form of overhead weight training for squats. I focused on strengthening my back by doing the plank everyday 3x/day for as long as I could hold the pose. I retreated from using any stairmaster or stepping equipment because I wanted my back to gain muscle and strength before attempting that type of pressure load on my back. This is something I decided to do in order to not push my discs out any further or have a reoccurrence. I continued to proceed with extra safety precautions as I had come to recognize that the healing process was one of a painful journey.

When tendons are torn and bone is chipped off

How I Do It

from a disc area, that area will heal with new tissue that is extremely tight and coarse. One must religiously stretch that area in order to gain back the flexibility and minimize the pain from it tightening up and pressing on the nerves.

To date, I will experience back pain or pressure depending on how long I sit or walk. However, I find that the healing has already taken place and that certain discs may currently have a degenerative cycle. However, I believe and have read that bone rebuilds within 6 months to a year; this all depends on your current health. I know that the pressure I feel is just simply the alignment of how the back muscles can put pressure on the bulging discs that have been left after these injuries. I was fortunate that my abdominal area and my overall health was great and I did not require any brace or any extensive physical therapy. In fact, after a few months, I decided that I already had the knowledge to take therapy into my own hands as one of my certifications is in fitness therapy.

Who would know better about your body than you? You need to take control of your mindset and seek whatever medical expertise you feel is needed in accordance to your injury. However, take note that healing starts with the mind and then the physical motion needs to be put in play in order to comeback from an injury and continue with your ADLs and your

How I Do It

fitness journey.

      Lastly, be patient with yourself-healing is a journey in itself. Take the time to heal properly so that you do not have any reoccurrences. And, most importantly, always listen to your body. You know your body better than anyone else.

How I Do It

Notes

How I Do It

Chapter Ten

TRAINING FOR ENDURANCE VS. STRENGTH

Endurance (aerobic) exercise requires more discipline in that your energy requirements are going to be far greater than strength (anaerobic) exercise. The refueling of energy stores becomes very critical for this type of training. Your carbohydrates become your life-saver!

For example, when I have planned on partaking in an endurance event like a marathon; I will include glucosamine into my diet a few months prior to training. I will make certain to take all my vitamins, eat approximately 70% of complex carbohydrates and provide myself with 2 days within a week for rest from running. I will train running 3x/wk. for 2 months indoor and then I will just "go for it". I challenge myself by running the marathon on a treadmill (indoors) with bathroom breaks only every hour. I have completed them in approximately 4:20 timeframe. During the marathon, I have used medication like ibuprofen or tylenol for hurting joints.

Further, I have never suffered an injury during training or while running a marathon. The fact is, my

How I Do It

body is already conditioned due to the fitness lifestyle I lead, and therefore 2 months or so are enough for me to expand my lungs enough to be able to sustain a run for 26.2 miles.

However, since I have coached people in running who are not in good physical condition to do so, my recommendations are based on that individual's fitness assessment. A thorough fitness evaluation is needed in order to properly approximate what one given individual should or should not do. Having said that, if your body is in a conditioned state that is use to working out for endurance and some strength 5 days a week, your attempt at running and finishing a race is quite good. However, if the opposite is true, the attempt may prove unsuccessful if you do not possess the agility, stamina, cardiovascular and muscular strength.

Therefore, if you are seriously thinking about running a race whether it is short or long distance; get a proper fitness evaluation in order to begin to understand what your training plan should incorporate. For example, if you have a weight issue, losing weight first is highly recommended as running takes a pounding on your joints especially your back. **(Consider walking incline on a treadmill or using a stairmaster to increase your heartrate to lose weight).** It is preferable to consider running a race when your weight is within your desired weight class.

How I Do It

The following is an example of a training plan that I designed for myself when I have run my marathons. This is my **8 week marathon training plan.**

Week	Mon	Wed	Sat	Total
1	4	4	8	16
2	4	5	10	19
3	4	6	11	21
4	5	5	8	18
5	6	6	10	22
6	6	6	10	22
7	8	rest	10	18
8	walk 4	walk 2	rest	run 26.2/32.2

I, personally envision myself running another marathon at some point because I love the serotonin rush I feel during and especially after a run. However, I prefer to exercise a bit more gently and with as little as possible stress during my perimenopausal years.

Strength training also referred to anaerobic is the resistance training on your muscular physique. It requires the proper rest and dedication as endurance

How I Do It

training however the restoring of energy fuels is less than the endurance athlete. As an anaerobic athlete, you should not partake in doing too much aerobic exercise if you are trying to build muscle mass. I basically will train a particular bodypart once a week in order to allow it the recovery and rebuilding timeframe. I will do a 2day/1dayoff routine and may interject some aerobic exercise to build my legs. I am careful to not over perform this activity as it will prove to be counteractive causing catabolism due to overtraining. It will most certainly sabotage my growth efforts.

Finally, both types of training require the proper supplementation and rest to allow the body to recover so that you can perform the sport to its maximum capability and achieve the best results.

How I Do It

Notes

How I Do It

Chapter Eleven

TRAINING PLATEAUS

Variation in training is very important in order to continue the evolution of change in your body. I believe the more your body has gotten accustomed to specific methods of training, it requires more of a challenge thus having to add diversity to your training plan-rule of adaptation. I have found that the traditional 4 to 6 weeks of training with the same routine is something that an avid fitness enthusiast would, more than likely, need to alter in order to see changes in the body. The 8 muscle groups (Shoulder, Chest, Trapezius, Arms, Forearms, Back, Abdominals and Legs) will require some more diversification training methods.

For example, if your walking is always at ground/flat level, the muscles are not going to develop any further as you have adapted those muscles to your workout. Therefore, when you use a treadmill or go outside to walk-try elevating the treadmill or walking on an uphill slope. This will shock the body as well as give you a more full range of motion on the glutes, hamstrings; quads, and calves training. Remember take into consideration where you are at in your level of training. If you are a beginner, then the 4 to 6 week rule of one training

How I Do It

plan should, more than likely, be followed and thereafter switching on to another routine. For you beginners, take solace that your body is in automatic shock during your initial training and will begin to make immediate changes.

However, if you are like me and the body is well adapted to various routines and/or methods, then I would highly recommend the constant switching of training the muscle groups. For example, I may decide to do mountain climbers and step-ups to hit my glutes while on another day I will do leg kickbacks with a cable cord and dumbbell squats. I make sure that the body is always guessing what else is next in order to keep the muscular structure at a balance of strength. My belief is that if you keep the body guessing your next move on all muscle groups, it will continue to keep the body's strength in balance.

How I Do It

Notes

How I Do It

Chapter Twelve

DIFFERENT THEORIES OF FAT STORAGE

First, vitamin C has been known to help keep the body burning fat due to the rebuilding processes and restoration of the muscle structures. It is arguably said if you are going to take any vitamin at all, vitamin C should be the one of choice.

Second, consume a non-fat high glycemic protein shake after your workout. The purpose of using a high glycemic shake without any fat would be to get the protein into the cells as quickly as possible. Fat slows the digestion process and therefore slows the muscle recovery.

Third, more research has indicated that anything with sugar will cause an instant trigger to insulin levels causing the body to start the fat storage process. It is suggesting that regular fruit is probably not the best choice while honey in protein should be used instead for quick cell recovery.

Fourth, consume a protein shake with just water and not add any other product to it. The theory here is that your body's insulin level is sufficient to bring this nutrient to your cells without having to add anything else.

How I Do It

Fifth, the temperature change will either cause fat to decrease or increase. When the body is not going through its biological changes during the colder months; it begins to release fat due to the warmer temperature change as it has no real need to store the extra fat. However, during the colder months; it will try and hold on to fat in order to be able to meet the demands of the body due to temperature change.

Sixth, arguably the best option of all is to consume some form of fat in every meal in order for the body to release fat. If the body does not receive fat in a snack/meal, it will begin its process of fat storage for survival.

Seventh, overtraining will cause the body to overstress and increase body fat storage. This is the very reason why you need to rest and allow the body its recovery time. Otherwise, you are simply sabotaging your training efforts and your body will not be representative of your hard-earned work.

In my opinion, I think all these theories are correct. They apply based on your bodyfat and your present training plan, and therefore each individual may have a different outcome. For me, the high glycemic (e.g., bananas, mangos, orange juice) protein shake works well after a workout because I keep my bodyfat low. However, when I want a softer-not as

How I Do It

ripped physique; I increase my bodyfat by incorporating pumpkin muffins or all-bran muffins with a protein shake.

You see, my belief is that the fat storage process is going to be triggered irrespective of how much fat is in your body. According to health statistics, the obesity count is huge and that leads me to believe the aforementioned. If your body recognized that you had sufficient fat-it would not hold on to it and cause overweight. However, because fat is used in survival mode, the body loves to store it and utilize it last.

How I Do It

Notes

How I Do It

Chapter Thirteen

PERIMENOPAUSE YEARS - Keeping The Beauty and Sexy Alive

Outer beauty is what is most visual to the eye. It is that quality that causes us to seek the perfect face and body. However, when we recognize that there is no such thing as "perfect"; we begin to simply enhance what we were given to work with in life. There are simple truths to obtaining the best quality of beauty at the cheapest rate. That is, sleep at least 8 hours a night, drink lots of water approximately 2 ounces per pound of bodyweight; and supplement with what is arguably the greatest vitamin - Vitamin C. These three things can make a big difference in the body and face.

First, vitamin "C" serves as a necessary nutrient to healing the body in all bodily functions. Aside from the Sun, it is arguably the most powerful antioxidant. The potency of this vitamin allows the rebuilding of collagen in the body. It produces a healthier looking face by enhancing the skin with its powerful antioxidants.

Second, since our body is made up of about 60 to 80% water; it is therefore necessary to consume water in order for our bodily functions to run in the most of optimal ways. By decreasing water, you may lose water weight and lessen the appearance of cellulite; however your face will become frail-looking and any wrinkles will be more visible because the plumpness is gone. Water keeps things flowing, glowing and looking vibrant. It rebuilds muscles, bones; ligaments, arteries; etc. and therefore should be consumed regularly throughout the day. The RDA recommendation is about eight glasses a day. However, for me and my physical demands; I drink approximately 16 ounces of water with every snack or meal and sometimes even more. Water is also wonderful for digestion thus excreting all toxins in the body. *Note: During cooler months, let the water sit warm outside of the refrigerator as cold water may be hard to consume when not working out.*

Second, sleeping 8 hours a night can really restore the body to its homeostasis level considering that there are no ailments at bay. The body rebuilds itself during the resting period. It is said that we get totally new cells within three months and bones rebuild within 6 months or so. However, if the body is not resting-then it is stressing, as I like to call it. It takes these three major components to really get the best quality of beauty that you will receive without breaking the budget.

Other products I use for beauty are fish oil,

almonds, blueberries, strawberries, coconut oil, olive oil, calcium, B-complex, B6, B12, Biotin and Zinc. These products are ones that I use regularly (with the exception of Biotin and Zinc usage for very high stressful times only) in order to combat any obstacles from my working out. As we age, these supplements become more critical in order to sustain energy levels that allow us to do our ADLs.

Stress
For women, it becomes a greater challenge during the change of life years. This time period is probably one, if not, the most difficult time in a woman's life. It is a time when stress levels skyrocket because the body is in a state of great change. It is a time that most women begin to really focus on their life. For those of us that have not reached mind, body and soul balance; I believe this is the time that truly stamps these three in equilibrium. We begin to accept the past, present and what the future may hold.

I have come to a stage where unnecessary stress has no place in my life and therefore have taken on various relaxation methods to help me on this journey.

First, I take a nap or rest period throughout the day in order to balance my body's hormonal levels. There are also a variety of herbs that one can take in order to calm the nervous system. Those herbs are

How I Do It

melatonin, valerian root, passionflower, ginseng, kava root, lemon balm, chamomile, skullcap and others. However, keep in mind that herbs can be very powerful especially if you are already on some type of medication.

Second, meditation is another form of relaxation. Some people meditate in order to calm their nervous system and ready it for sleep. Others, like me use it to get in mind, body and soul in balance. This is one of the times I speak to my Higher Power. However, I find myself speaking with my Higher Power all day as I choose to live a life of internal peace in all areas of my life.

Third, stretching is another form of relaxation- it is a part of yoga and pilates. When you elongate your body through stretching, the muscles begin to relax and provide the release of tension along with resting the musculoskeletal structure. It can prove to be a helpful precursor to sleep as it provides the relaxation mode to the resting phase of sleep.

Fourth, in the colder months of the year, I use my Jacuzzi for relaxation and muscle tension. It is amazing the benefits a heated bath can have by the massaging effect on the muscles. This is probably my favorite form of relaxation.

Fifth, I will also use an inversion bed for

relaxation. This bed serves a number of benefits. It relaxes muscles and provides this feel good hormone (serotonin) to flow to one's head. The effects that one can get from the function of body inversion can prove to be quite relaxing.

Finally, for women in this change of life phase prescribed medications are available to help with insomnia during this time. However, I suggest you do everything possible in a holistic manner. If you have not already consulted with a licensed physician; then seek that practitioner's medical advice.

Energy
During the perimenopausal years, women definitely find their energy levels declining and whether your employment is at home or not, you will find that your nervous system may get short at times and unable to tolerate stressful situations. In addition, if you happen to workout-the demands on your body become much greater and the need to balance your hormones becomes more critical. I have found that B-Complex and/or B-6/B-12 along with vitamin C have helped me tremendously. The need for these supplements will vary depending on the strenuous level of my workouts or ADLs.

Facial, Neck and Body
Olive and coconut oil - I use these both combined every time I wash my face. I have found

How I Do It

that after rinsing my face with the warmest water and applying the aforementioned, I get a more rejuvenated look instead of closing the pours with cold water as I use to do. The warmest water will open up the pores and allow the moisturizer to seep into your skin. Do the same for your neck area. I have practiced this ritual for approximately 3 years and from my teenage years, I have always used cocoa butter on my face and no other type of cream. I also use cocoa butter regularly on my entire body every time I shower. I have been doing this for approximately 30 years. Further, when I focus on eliminating scarring tissue from a blemish; I just use coconut oil or 100% cocoa butter and sometimes vitamin E.

In addition, I sometimes use a honey/olive oil mask for approximately 1 hour around my face and under eyelids where wrinkles tend to become more prominent. There are also times when I will put honey with olive oil under eyelids overnight.

Botox is something I just explored a handful of times during this past year or so. I do not have any real wrinkles to speak of at the moment other than the ones under my eyelids that are more noticeable during my times of laughter. I felt that since my stress levels were elevating due to perimenopause; I would give it a try as a preventative treatment. Depending on my stress levels, I have found the treatment's lasting effect to vary and can be very short term. I find it to be very costly and do not know whether I will continue down this road. This is one of the main reasons why I decided to further diversify my workouts with more overall body training and lighter weights, thus lessening the stress on my body.

Exfoliate

For my face, I use coffee or brown sugar with my preferred facial soap (neutrogena) and a facial scrub. I rotate it in circular motion for 30 seconds to 2 minutes varying on how much old skin there is to remove. Afterwards, I rinse with warm water and apply the coconut oil/olive oil mix that I use daily. I will try and exfoliate once a week. As for my body, I just use soap and water.

Detoxify the Body

There are certainly many methods to detoxify your body. I use a variety of them when needed. Prunes are considered to be one of the highest detoxification fruits. On occasion, I will digest one or two depending on my nutrition plan. Lemons and warm water can also cleanse your systems, primarily the liver. This is probably a really good inexpensive treatment when on regular medication(s). As I indicated earlier, I do not really use flaxseed at my current stage in life-it's on rare occasion. My favorite is always drinking lots of water during the day. I basically have only coffee in the morning and, thereafter; it is pure water for me with rare instances of decaffeinated coffee or tea. You will find that as the body releases toxins due to detoxification, the skin looks more vibrant and youthful.

Reduce Bloating During Menstrual Cycle

Reduce the sodium in meals a couple days prior to getting your period to reduce bloating but do not stop drinking water. This will help the bloating effect as well as inflammation. Aloe Vera is a very good anti-inflammatory along with fish oil and flax seed. Also try and stay away from other foods like beans, cauliflower, broccoli, sugars and refined carbohydrates as they can also contribute to bloating.

Mouth & Teeth Hygiene

I have never had my teeth whitened but what I have used regularly for about 10 years is hydrogen peroxide and toothpaste. First, I gargle with mouthwash, then gargle with peroxide for about a minute and thereafter brush thoroughly. I do this at least two times daily (morning and before bed). I floss every time I eat-that is about 6 times daily.

I have found that once you have crowns or spacing between some of your molars; the irritation of foods in those areas can cause inflammation among other bacterial infections. It is best to stay safe and keep the mouth as clean as much as possible.

If my gums happen to get irritated, I gargle

How I Do It

with sea salt warm water every hour to reduce the swelling. This rarely happens to me as I try to eat clean but on those rare occasions where I may snack on popcorn, hard crackers or some form of tortilla chip; it usually causes this irritation.

Antioxidant Foods
There are quite a number of antioxidant foods that you can eat to slow down the aging process. I will list the foods that I eat regularly and that work well thus far during my beginning stages of perimenopause.

- Dark Organic Chocolate w/ or without Almonds at highest Cocoa percentage.
- Roasted Peanuts, Oatmeal, Blueberries, Strawberries, Papaya, Soy milk, Soynut Butter, Broccoli, Spinach, Red Grapes, Whole Grains, Red Kidney Beans and Black Beans.

I eat dark organic chocolate (preferably 90% cocoa) as the cocoa appears to have anti-aging and anti-inflammatory properties. Also, cocoa is a good source of the minerals magnesium, sulphur, calcium, iron, zinc, copper, potassium, and manganese; plus some of the B Vitamins.

Sunshine
The Sun is arguably the most powerful antioxidant for the body. Based on research, the Sun

How I Do It

provides health for all bodily organs and healing disorders like arthritis, anxiety, depression, etc. For me, the benefits have outweighed the negatives in causing wrinkles. The wrinkles under my eyes are basically from laughter and lack of fat and not necessarily from the Sun. They are really only noticeable during times of laughter. Other than that, the Sun has kept my skin looking vibrant and youthful as it provides the release of toxins through its energy flow.

In fact, studies have shown that it is the sunscreen that contains the toxins that seep into our skin. Nevertheless, this past year I started using sunscreen regularly while outdoors to evaluate whether it proves to minimize or eliminate the formation of wrinkles. In the past, I have only used sunscreen on rare occasions where I may be out for long durations with direct sun exposure. I try and allow daily exposure to the Sun for a minimum of 20 minutes to 1 hour without any sunscreen. In the Fall and Winter months, I will meditate by my window and allow the Sun to enter through my eyes without looking directly at the Sun. It flows its energy through the eyes and serves as a key leader in the creation of vitamin D. This vitamin is key to providing a soothing and relaxing state in the body. If there is no Sun out, I will either opt to further supplement with additional Vitamin D or drink milk (nonfat or soy).

How I Do It

Notes

How I Do It

Chapter Fourteen

GENETICS - FIBER TYPE 1 OR TYPE II

The components of the human physiology play a big role in determining better muscle building genetics. The most obvious would be that of your natural testosterone levels. The other major component would be your muscle type fiber makeup. There is a different percentage of either slow-twitch type I or fast-twitch type II fibers that varies between muscles and individuals. The type of fiber varies in their functions of the muscle building process. Slow-twitch fiber type I individuals do better in endurance but do not have the great capability of hypertrophy. Fast-twitch fiber type II individuals are not very good at endurance as they fatigue quickly but have greater capabilities in hypertrophy than slow-twitch fiber type I individuals.

Research has shown that if you follow some of the suggested; testosterone levels can be maintained or even increase.

1) Exercise But Do Not Overtrain - Too much training especially cardiovascular will cause the body to stress thus increasing cortisol and lowering testosterone.

How I Do It

2) High Fat Diet - Your Omega-3's, monounsaturated and even saturated fats in diet, have all shown to increase testosterone levels.

3) Zinc and Vitamin B6 - This mineral and vitamin seem to work well with athletes in maintaining healthy testosterone levels.

4) Quality Consistent Sleep - Your body balances and recuperates your hormone levels while sleeping and therefore it is recommended that you get at least 8 hours of consecutive sleep.

5) Long Term Dieting - If you are in a calorie deficit, your testosterone levels will decrease due to the release of cortisol. In addition, you will not be as energetic due to the lowering of hormones in your thyroid.

6) Medication - Always evaluate the type of medications you are taking as they may play a role in lowering your testosterone levels.

7) Warm Weather - There are studies that have shown that with cooler weather, testosterone levels drop and therefore warmer weather especially throughout the year helps in maintaining testosterone levels.

How I Do It

Notes

Chapter Fifteen

FOODS

These are some of the meals I have throughout my day and are not in any particular order based on physique's appearance. That has been noted in the Nutrition Chapter what and how I eat in order to get the type of appearance in my physique. I do want to point out again that I do drink a cup or two of coffee in the morning each day. I do not believe in giving up my caffeine as it helps with digestion and energy. Thereafter I drink water for the rest of the day with, on occasion, a cup of decaffeinated tea or coffee aside from some of the shakes noted below.

Shakes

Note: With most of my shakes (mostly whey and sometimes soy protein), I have started adding fiber to them as oppose to flaxseed. Again, I am currently exploring the estrogenic effect without making much use of flaxseed in my current perimenopausal stage.

- Spinach Protein Shake - orange juice, cup of spinach, water and 10gms of protein (optional celery and/or pineapple)
- Banana Protein Shake w/ small banana

How I Do It

(sometimes take fish oil if prior to workout)
- Strawberry/Blueberry Protein Shake w/ real strawberries and blueberries
- Mango Protein Shake w/ real mango
- Soy Shake - Soymilk, water and 10gms of protein
- Soy Almond Shake - Soymilk, handful of almonds and water
- Bran or Pumpkin Muffin and Protein Shake
- Papaya Protein Shake
- Dark Chocolate Protein Shake - I will use a 1 1/2 servings of 90% DC with protein and splendid

Snacks
- Whole Grain Bread with Soynut Butter or Organic Peanut Butter w/or Sugar-free Jelly/Jam
- Sardines with Spinach
- Yogurt-low in sugar or sugar-free (Greek Yogurt or Organic)-sometimes add fiber, berries and granola to it.
- Dark Organic Chocolate w/ almonds or peanut butter or soynut butter
- Handful of unsalted nuts (e.g., roasted peanuts, raw almonds, walnuts)
- Apple/Banana with peanut butter/soynut butter

Meals
- Protein Pancakes made with olive-oil
- Egg White Cheese Wrap - 1 whole egg and 3 egg whites with light cheese on a whole grain wrap
- Egg White Omelette w Spinach made with olive

How I Do It

oil
- Oatmeal with or without Soy Milk
- High Fiber Cereal
- Chicken with Olive Oil-Wrap - chicken, celery bits, spinach and light cheese
- Tilapia with Brown Rice - Tilapia (green peas, broccoli or spinach), brown rice, balsamic, or spray herb
- Grilled Salmon - Salmon with asparagus (with or without brown rice (or) 1 slice whole grain bread)
- Tuna Melt - Tuna, light cheese or nonfat cheese, spinach and 1 slice of whole grain bread
- Tuna Olive-Oil Wrap - Tuna, spinach, light cheese and olive-oil wrap
- Grilled Tomato Wrap - Tomato, olive-oil wrap, light cheese and spray with olive-oil or 1 tbspn of organic olive oil
- Grilled Chicken Tomato - Chicken, tomato, light cheese and 1 tbspn of olive-oil or olive-oil cooking spray
- Bean Burritos w/ onions, green peppers, rice and light cheese
- Herb-crusted Halibut, Asparagus & Brown Rice
- Pizza with Tuna or any other lean protein
- Scallops, Zucchini, Brown Rice, Green Peppers
- Variety of Soups (e.g., Lentil, Black Beans, Lima Beans, Chicken, Tuna) with squash, celery, onions, carrots(optional) & nuts(optional)
- Variety of Salads (e.g., Chicken, Tuna, Scallops, Shrimp) with avocado, nuts, mandarins and

How I Do It

balsamic vinegar

How I Do It

Notes

How I Do It

Chapter Sixteen

HANDLING HOLIDAY FESTIVITIES

What I basically do for any holiday (e.g., 4th of July, Thanksgiving, New Year's) is I prepare myself for the inevitable. I know there is going to be plenty of sinful treats and I want to make certain to enjoy some of those treats. Therefore, I begin by making certain that I have begun to incorporate more strength training a week prior to the holiday event. **I do this in order to get my muscles really hungry** for those carbohydrates that I will, more than likely, want to enjoy.

I will also incorporate some of the following to my pre-party festivity:

- Bring a protein bottle just in case I stay longer than planned;
- Drink lots of H20 while at festivity;
- Eat a small meal before heading to the event;
- Bring along some healthy snacks in bag/purse in case there isn't anything healthy on the menu;
- I rarely ever drink but might have a glass of wine for New Year's or so;
- I brown bag some of the food/treats for later eats. I will have them during the week so I do not feel

How I Do It

as if I missed out on some of my favorite sinful treats.

How I Do It

Notes

How I Do It

Glossary of Terms

A

Abductor Muscle - Any muscle used to pull a body part away from the midline of the body.
Abs - Slang for abdominal muscles.
Adaptation - The degree of adjustment of the body in fitness.
ADLs - Activities of Daily Living.
Adductor Muscle - a muscle that draws a body part inward towards the median line.
Aerobic - Exercise using oxygen.
Amino Acids - The building blocks of protein.
Anaerobic - Exercise without using oxygen.
Antioxidants - These are certain minerals, vitamins and nutrients that protect the body against free-radicals.
Anterior - The front.
Arthritis - Inflammation of the joints which causes pain, stiffness and limitation of motion.
Atrophy - A decrease in size of muscle.

B

Biceps - The prominent muscle in the front of the arm.
Biotin - Member of the B complex vitamin that is essential for metabolizing fat, protein, vitamin C and B12.
Blood - The fluid which circulates through the heart, arteries, veins and capillaries.

How I Do It

BMR (Basal Metabolic Rate) - The rate that the body burns calories while at complete rest over a 24 period.
Bodyfat - The percentage of fat in the body.

C

Calcium - A vital mineral that is most abundant in the body forming bones, teeth, muscle growth, muscle contraction, the regulation of nutrient passage in/out of cells and nerve transmissions.
Carbohydrates - One of the three basic nutrients (with proteins and fats being the others). They are the most important source of energy for your body.
Cellulite - Adipose fat tissue.
Collagen - The most abundant protein in the body that forms tough connective tissue.
Concentric-Is the movement where the muscle shortens during its contraction.
Cycle - Refers to a female's menstruation.

D

Deltoids - It is the large triangular muscle of the shoulder that serves to be the prime mover in all arm elevation movements.
Dumbbell - It is a weight used for exercising that varies in shape but consists of a handle with two weighted objects on either end. Some of these are automatically built together while others allow for adding weighted objects to either end.

E

Endorphins - Brain chemicals that ease or suppress pain. These are considered natural painkillers.
Endurance - The capacity to continue physical

performance over a given period of time.
Energy - The capacity to produce function of the bodily organs towards performance.
Exercise - The physical exertion of the body for fitness and/or activities of daily living.

F

Fast-Twitch Fiber Type II - Type II muscles are good for short-term activities that require lots of energy because it is good at generating power. However, this type of muscle fatigues quickly due to anaerobic metabolism.
Fiber - The part of a plant food that is associated with assisting in the digestion process.
Fitness - The state of well-being at optimum levels of strength, flexibility and cardiovascular capacity.
Fitness Assessment/Evaluation - The measurement of levels in fitness.

G

Glucosamine - A natural compound that is found in healthy cartilage. It is available as a supplement in liquid or tablet form.
Glycemic Index - A rating system that indicates the speed at which carbohydrates are processed into glucose by body.

H

Heartrate - The number of times your heart beats in a minute.
Herbs - A part of a plant that may be used as a medical treatment, nutrient, food seasoning or dye.
Homeostatis - The tendency of the body to maintain

How I Do It

its internal systems in balance.

Hormones - Chemical substances that originate in an organ, gland, or body part and are transmitted by the blood to affect the functions of the body.

Hypertrophy - An increase in size of muscle.

I

Inflammation - Is the swelling due to a bodily function that is typically characterized by pain, heat, bloating and redness.

Intensity - The rate of performing work.

J

Joints - Formed where two bones come together.

~K~

L

Lats (Latissimus Dorsi) - The large back muscles that are prime movers for adduction, extension and hyperextension of shoulder joint.

M

Menopause - The time when a women stops her menstruation for a consecutive period of 12 months.

Minerals - Any of a class of substances occurring in nature, usually comprising inorganic substances, as quartz or feldspar, of definite chemical.

Muscle - Tissue consisting of fibers organized into bands or bundles that contract to perform bodily movement.

Muscle Group - Muscles that act together at same joint to produce a movement.

N

Nutrient - The elements and compounds of a food

How I Do It

that can be used by the body to build and maintain itself and to produce energy.

Nutrition - The use of nutrients.

O

Oblique - A very large muscle running down the side of your body. It extends from your ribs into your abdomen.

Osteoarthritis - The most common joint disorder. The chronic disease causes the cushioning (cartilage) between the bone joints to wear away, leading to pain and stiffness.

Overtraining - Excessive training typically in the strength and endurance athlete.

P

Physiological - Characteristic of or appropriate to an organism's healthy or normal functioning.

Posterior - The back.

Protein - Complex substances present in living organisms. They comprise of 70% skin, 80% muscles and 90% of dry weight of blood.

Q

Quadriceps - A muscle group in front of the thigh that connects to tendon that surrounds the kneecap and attaches to the tibia (lower leg bone).

R

Repetition - A completed exercise movement.

Resistance -The force of which a muscle is required to work against.

Reverse flyes - Exercise that target the rear or posterior deltoids in similar fashion to lateral raises.

How I Do It

S

Saturated Fat - Dietary source found in primarily animal sources and is a contributor to blood cholesterol levels and linked to increase heart disease.
Set - A group of repetitions of an exercise movement done consecutively.
Skeletal Muscle - Muscle that attaches to skeletal structure and causes body movement by a shortening or pulling action against its bony attachment.
Slow-Twitch Fiber Type I - A muscle fiber type that contracts slowly and is used in moderate-intensity or endurance exercise.
Squats - An upper leg and hip exercise performed with a pair of dumbbells hanging on either side of body or a barbell resting on shoulders.
Strength Training -Using resistance weight training to build max muscle force is the traditional way of defining the practice of strength training.
Stress - The general physical and psychological response of an individual to any real or perceived adverse stimulus, internal or external, that tends to disturb the individual's homeostatis.
Sucrose - A sweet disaccharide that occurs naturally in most land plants and is the simple carbohydrate obtained from sugarcane, sugar beet and other sources.
Supine - Lying on the back with face upward.
Supplements - A product which helps to fulfill

certain needs of the body which cannot be completed or provided by the body.

T

Testosterone - The sex hormone that predominates in the male body and is involved in the hypertrophy of muscle.

Training - The undergoing of repeated stresses and recovery periods on the body for growth to handle such stresses.

Triceps - The muscles on the back of the upper arm which are prime movers for extending the elbow.

U

Unsaturated Fat - Is a fat or fatty acid in which there is at least one double bond within the fatty acid chain.

V

Vitamin - Is an organic compound required as a nutrient in tiny amounts by an organism.

Vitamin B Complex - Made up of vitamins (B_1, B_2, B_3 B5, B6, B7, B9 & B12).

Vitamin B6 - Is a water-soluble vitamin and is part of the vitamin B complex group.

Vitamin B12 - Is a water soluble vitamin with a key role in the normal functioning of the brain and nervous system.

Vitamin C - Is an essential nutrient for humans and certain other animal species, in which it functions as a vitamin.

Vitamin D - Is a group of fat-soluble secosteroids, the two major physiologically relevant forms of which are vitamin D_2 and vitamin D_3.

How I Do It

W

Warm-up - The gradual increase in the intensity of exercise that allow bodily processes to prepare for greater energy outputs thus increasing the rise of body temperature.

Weight Training - Exercise that use resistance movements to build strength.

~X,Y~

Z

Zinc - Is an essential mineral.

Made in the USA
Columbia, SC
08 December 2018